YOUR KNOWLEDGE HAS VALUE

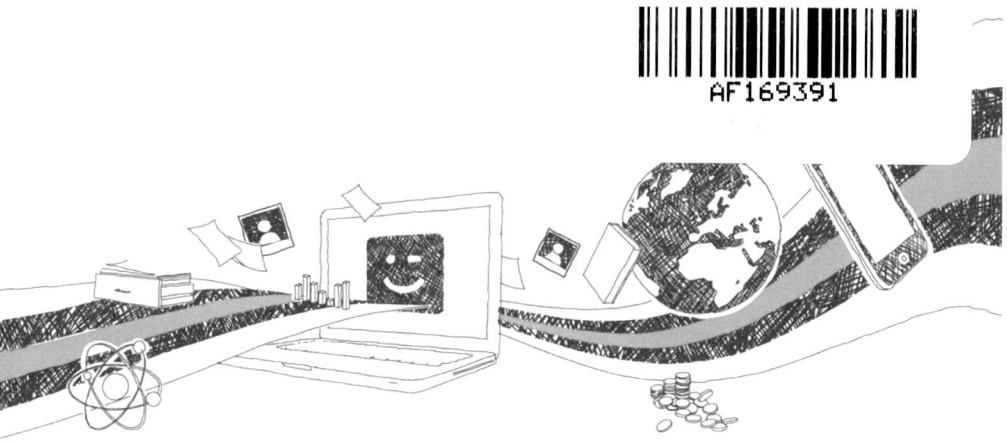

- We will publish your bachelor's and master's thesis, essays and papers

- Your own eBook and book - sold worldwide in all relevant shops

- Earn money with each sale

Upload your text at www.GRIN.com
and publish for free

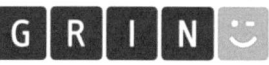

Bibliographic information published by the German National Library:

The German National Library lists this publication in the National Bibliography; detailed bibliographic data are available on the Internet at http://dnb.dnb.de .

This book is copyright material and must not be copied, reproduced, transferred, distributed, leased, licensed or publicly performed or used in any way except as specifically permitted in writing by the publishers, as allowed under the terms and conditions under which it was purchased or as strictly permitted by applicable copyright law. Any unauthorized distribution or use of this text may be a direct infringement of the author s and publisher s rights and those responsible may be liable in law accordingly.

Imprint:

Copyright © 2018 GRIN Verlag
Print and binding: Books on Demand GmbH, Norderstedt Germany
ISBN: 9783668638402

This book at GRIN:

https://www.grin.com/document/411947

Patrick Kimuyu

Understanding Hypoactive Sexual Desire Disorder

GRIN Verlag

GRIN - Your knowledge has value

Since its foundation in 1998, GRIN has specialized in publishing academic texts by students, college teachers and other academics as e-book and printed book. The website www.grin.com is an ideal platform for presenting term papers, final papers, scientific essays, dissertations and specialist books.

Visit us on the internet:

http://www.grin.com/

http://www.facebook.com/grincom

http://www.twitter.com/grin_com

Understanding Hypoactive Sexual Desire Disorder

Name: Patrick Kimuyu

Introduction

In retrospect, sexual disorders have a significant impact on an individual's quality of life (Lindau et al., 2007). It is also apparent that these disorders bear immense significance to the clinical practice (Kingsberg, 2011). Despite their impact, most physicians do not seem to be interested to engage in extensive discussion with patients regarding sexual desire problems. This phenomenon is, probably, attributable to several reasons including time constraints, lack of efficient therapeutic interventions and insufficient knowledge. One of the most debilitating sexual desire disorders is hypoactive sexual desire disorder (HSDD). HSDD is also known as inhibited sexual desire (ISD) (Rice & Kim, 2015). HSDD is characterized by decreased or absence of desire for sexual activity and sexual fantasies which causes interpersonal difficulties, as well as personal distress (Nappi et al., 2010). In some circumstances, the diagnosis of HSDD exhibits co-morbidity to an underlying sexual dysfunction. However, this disorder is not exclusively attributed to the effects of any substance, pathology or another psychiatric disorder (Basson et al., 2010). Even though some clinical experts have hypothesized the causes of HSDD to be associated with biological imbalances, the pathophysiology of this disorder remains unknown. As such, efforts to develop a comprehensive treatment and management strategies have not achieved remarkable success. Therefore, this literature review aims at providing an overview of HSDD.

Epidemiology

Epidemiological trends of HSDD exhibit gender inequalities in which women are more affected than men. Research studies indicate that sexual dysfunction occurs at a higher magnitude among women than men. This phenomenon is evidenced by several studies which have investigated sexuality. According to Gingell et al. (2005), an estimated 13% to 28% of men in the US were experiencing low sexual desire problems as compared to 26% to 43% among women by

2005. Overall, it is estimated that up to 25% of women in the US are suffering from HSDD (Warnock, 2002). Evidence the high prevalence of HSDD among women was reaffirmed by the findings of the WISHes (Women's International Study of Health and Sexuality) which showed that 24% to 36% of women experienced low sexual desire (Barton, Koochaki, Leiblum, Rodenberg & Rosen, 2006). In another prospective study, the prevalence of HSDD among women was found to vary with age in which middle-aged women (45 to 64 years) have the highest prevalence of 12.3%, whereas those aged 18 to 44 years and older than 65 years have prevalence rates of 8.9% and 7.4%, respectively (Shifren, Monz, Russo, Segreti & Johannes, 2008). On the other hand, the prevalence of HSDD seems to increase with aging which causes a significant decrease in sexual desire among men and women. A prospective study carried out by Brotto (2010) showed that only 4% of women had sexual desire at the age of 67 years compared to 14% among men. This was contrary to the trends in 16 to 24 years of age in which 72% and 50% sexual desire were reported in men and women, respectively. Overall, it is reported that the prevalence of HSDD is similar in the US and UK, especially with reference to the prevalence among women in which 1 in every 10 women is experiencing HSDD (Clayton, 2010).

History of HSDD

Over the decades, definition and classification of sexual dysfunction has been advancing year-by-year due to extensive scientific inquiry on sexual desire problems within the global population. Initially, two sexual dysfunction; impotence among men and frigidity among women, were recognized. These dysfunctions were attributable to the biological functions of the genitals. Following the description of these sexual dysfunctions in 1970, sex therapy became the mainstay for the management of low sexual desire. Despite the recognition of low sexual desire in the early 1970s, this condition was not categorized as one of the main sexual dysfunction until 1977 when

Harold Lief and Helen Singer Kaplan described it independently. This is where the terms 'Hypoactive sexual Desire' and 'Inhibited Sexual Desire' emerged as the description for HSDD by Kaplan and Lief, respectively (Irvine, 2005).

It was from the work of Leif and Kaplan, sex therapists that led to the inclusion of HSDD into the Diagnostic and Statistical Manual of Mental Disorders (DSM). As such, HSDD appeared in DSM-III which was published in 1980. This marked the beginning of a universal diagnosis of HSDD to avoid misdiagnosis attributable to cultural differences. Ordinarily, low sexual desire is defined from different social contexts in which some cultures do not consider it as a sexual dysfunction, but rather a normal condition. It is also apparent that the magnitude of low sexual desire varies across cultures. For instance, it is reported that American populations exhibit a higher sexual desire compared to Asian populations (Brotto, Chik, Ryder, Gorzalka & Seal, 2005).

Later in 1987, the revision of DSM-III (DSM-II-R) created two subdivisions of ISD: Sexual Aversion Disorder (SAD) and Hypoactive Sexual Desire Disorder (HSDD). Further revision on the DSM-III-R criterion led to the inclusion of personal distress as part of HSDD diagnosis as described in DSM-IV of 1994 (Irvine, 2005). Recently in 2013, DSM-5 split HSDD into two subsets: female sexual interest/arousal disorder and male hypoactive sexual desire disorder. The scientific rationale for creating this distinction was based on the fact that the intensity and frequency of sexual desire vary between men and women (American Psychiatric Association, 2013a).

Etiology of HSDD

Even though the pathophysiology of HSDD remains a mystery, it etiology is clearly understood. Clayton (2010) reports that the causes of HSDD are multifactorial in which an array of causative and contributing factors exist. Clinical studies suggest interplay among psychological, neurological and hormonal factors which is responsible for the balance of excitatory and inhibitory activities in the brain. Ordinarily, dopamine, testosterone, progesterone, and estrogen are considered as the main excitatory factors which are responsible for sexual desire. On the other hand, prolactin and serotonin are antagonistic to excitatory factors; thus, they enhance inhibitory activity (Clayton, 2010). In general, testosterone and estrogen deficiencies are considered as the principle causes of HSDD.

Low Testosterone

Low testosterone has been hypothesized as one of the main underlying causes of HSDD. Biologically, testosterone plays integral roles in controlling sexual behavior, as well as exciting sexual activity. Overall, testosterone is responsible for genital engorgement in both men and women. It is also controls clitoral and vaginal physiology including lubrication and sensation (Brundu et al., 2003). As such, it is apparent that testosterone controls the physiology of genitals in humans. Therefore, low production or lack of it has been found to be associated with physiological consequences. According to Davis and Tran (2001), lack of testosterone leads to low libido, as well as decreased sexual pleasure. This explains why menopausal women experience low sexual desire compared to young women due to the decline of testosterone production.

Low Estrogen

Lack of estrogen has been identified as another cause of HSDD. Ordinarily, estrogen is responsible for sexual responsiveness. It also controls the physiology of the female genitalia through lubrication. In the case of HSDD, estrogen deficiency leads to vaginal dryness, mood changes and hot flashes. Vaginal dryness is usually responsible for painful intercourse which affects sexual pleasure and receptivity. Moreover, lack of estrogen causes imbalance of inhibitors which regulate sexual response cycle such as selective serotonin reuptake inhibitors (Nappi et al.,

2010). For instance, it leads to sleep disturbances; thus decreasing the quality of life as a result of personal distress.

Other Causes of HSDD

In retrospect, it is apparent that hormonal changes are not the only cause of HSDD. It has also been found to be caused by other medical conditions such as Cushing's disease, diabetes mellitus, menopause, Addison's disease, stroke, renal failure, heart disease, and hypothyroidism (Abdallah & Simon, 2007). Other causes include hormonal imbalances during lactation and pregnancy. Moreover, medications, especially those which inhibit dopamine release or enhance prolactin release have been found to cause HSDD (Stahl, 2000).

Risk Factors

HSDD, like most disorders has risk factors which underlie its onset in some circumstances. These risk factors increase the individual's susceptibility to the disorder. Some of the main risk factors which have been investigated extensively include relationship factors and aging. Ordinarily, relationships have immense impacts on an individual's social behavior, including sexuality. Evidence shows that sexual distress causes depression, especially in strained relationships. This aspect is not often in relationships where efficient communication of sexual needs exist (Hayes et al., 2008). Therefore, it is imperative that depression among partners or couples is the culprit for low sexual desire.

On the other hand, aging has been found to increase the risk of HSDD. Young adults experience high sexual desire compared to the aged. This is attributable to physiological changes during aging including hormonal deficiencies as it is the case in menopause. However, evidence shows that young adults experience more distress due to low sexual desire than old adults. These phenomena explain why the prevalence of HSDD tends to be constant over time (Hayes et al., 2007).

Diagnosis of HSDD

In practice, diagnosis for HSDD is based on DSM-5 criteria. This diagnosis approach defines the symptoms which must be present in both men and women. However, physicians are required to judge the occurrence of HSDD based on the patient's cultural context and age (Brotto, 2010). In men, the diagnosis for male hypoactive sexual desire disorder is based on criteria A1-6, B and C. Overall, the presence of absence or reduced sexual fantasies, interest in sexual activity, lack of receptivity, and sexual pleasure/excitement suggests HSDD. In addition, failure to get sexually aroused without stimulation, absence of genital changes during intercourse, presence of distress, and exclusion of another Axis I disorder confirm HSDD diagnosis (American Psychiatric Association, 2013a).

On the other hand, diagnosis of HSDD in women is governed by the hallmark features which are defined under DSM-5 with respect to female sexual interest/arousal disorder. According to the American Psychiatric Association (2013b), the occurrence of at least three of the defined hallmark features confirms HSDD diagnosis. These symptoms include lack or reduced interest in sexual intercourse, external or internal erotic stimuli, response to sexual initiation, sexual thoughts, and reduced or absence of genital sensations. Overall, both situations require the existence of lifelong absences of sexual desire. In DSM-5, unlike the previous version (DSM-IV), frequency and duration requirements are defined. First, diagnosis of HSDD should be confirmed after a minimum duration of six months. Second, the hallmark presentation features must be evident in 75% to 100% of the diagnosis period (IsHak & Tobia, 2013).

Co-morbidity

In most cases, HSDD co-occur with other sexual dysfunctions. This explains why this disorder is often misdiagnosed. For instance, erectile dysfunction in men may underlie the occurrence of HSDD (Montgomery, 2008). Vaginismus in women reflects similar conditions. Moreover, HSDD is often masked by dyspareunia.

Interventions/Treatment

In practice, the management of HSDD encompasses some complexities which are attributable to the underlying pathophysiology, especially with respect to its causes and contributing factors. As such, interventions focus on addressing the consequences of the disorder and improving the quality of life. Current interventions include psychotherapy and pharmacotherapy. Medications can be used alone or combined with psychotherapy.

Psychotherapy

Over the decades, psychotherapy has been the touchstone in the management of sexual desire disorders. The scientific rationale for the widespread popularity of psychotherapy is based on the fact that sexual dysfunction arises from unsolved developmental conflicts (Montgomery, 2008).

Cognitive behavioral therapy (CBT)

CBT focuses on addressing depression and anxiety to reduce personal distress. In this context, CBT has been found to be effective in controlling sexual behaviors that may lead to low sexual desire. Some of the key aspects addressed by CBT are unrealistic sexual expectations and dysfunctional thoughts. In practice, most CBT sessions involve both partners (Trudel et al., 2001).

Sex Therapy

Sex therapy has a long history in the treatment of sexual dysfunctions. This therapy aims at enhancing sexual response cycle through improved communication within a relationship, primarily on sexual needs of the partners. From a psychodynamic lens, the combination of psychoanalytic strategies with sex therapy bears appreciable outcomes (Sadock & Sadock, 2003).

Pharmacotherapy

Despite the lack of curative agents for the treatment of HSDD, some agents have been in use for the management of HSDD.

Hormone Therapy

Hormone therapy involves the use of hormonal substances to address hormonal deficiencies. Some of the most beneficial hormone therapies which are used for the treatment of HSDD include androgen therapy, estrogen-progestin therapy, estrogen therapy, testosterone therapy, and tibolone therapy (Nappi et al., 2010).

Other Medications

Some medications have also been found to be useful in increasing sexual desire in HSDD patients. These medications include methylphenidate, amphetamine and bupropion (Montgomery, 2008). Recently, flibanserin was approved by the US FDA, exclusively for the treatment of HSDD. However, the use of this drug is somehow controversial due to its contraindications. First, it has high alcohol interaction in both men and women. Second, it has some adverse side effects including CNS depression (Hylton et al., 2016).

Conclusion

Conclusively, HSDD has emerged as clinically significant sexual dysfunction. It impacts on the clinical practice, as well as, the individual's quality of life. This implies that appropriate diagnosis and treatment is paramount in reducing its burden. However, effective diagnosis is impaired by co-morbidity which is the principal cause of misdiagnosis. Nevertheless, the recently published DSM-5 seems to improve HSDD diagnosis. On the other hand, extensive research on the underlying pathophysiology of HSDD has led to the development of efficient intervention approaches. Of the major advances in HSDD management is the approval of flibanserin by FDA. Moreover, psychotherapy has expanded to include psychoanalytic and psychodynamic perspectives.

References

Abdallah, R. T., & Simon, J. A. (2007). Testosterone therapy in women: its role in the management of hypoactive sexual desire disorder. *Int J Impotence Res.*, *19*, 458–463

American Psychiatric Association. (2013a). *Male hypoactive sexual desire disorder, 302.71 (F52.0). Diagnostic and statistical manual of mental disorders,* (5th ed). Arlington, VA: American Psychiatric Publishing.

American Psychiatric Association. (2013b). *Female sexual interest/arousal disorder, 302.72 (F52.22). Diagnostic and statistical manual of mental disorders* (5th ed). Arlington, VA: American Psychiatric Publishing.

Barton, I., Koochaki, P., Leiblum, S., Rodenberg, C., & Rosen, R. (2006). Hypoactive sexual desire disorder in postmenopausal women: U.S. results from the women's international study of health and sexuality (WISHeS). *Menopause, 13*(1), 46–56.

Basson, R., Berman, J., Burnett, A., Derogatis, L., Ferguson, D., Fourcroy, J.,…Whipple, B. (2010). Summary of the recommendations of sexual dysfunction in women. *J Sex Med.*, *7*(1 Pt 2), 314–326.

Brotto, L. A. (2010). The DSM diagnostic criteria for hypoactive sexual desire disorder in men. *J Sex Med.*, *7*, 2015–2030. DOI: 10.1111/j.1743-6109.2010.01860.x

Brotto, L. A., Chik, H. M., Ryder, A. G., Gorzalka, B. B., & Seal, B (2005). Acculturation and sexual function in Asian women. *Archives of Sexual Behavior, 34*(6), 613–626. DOI: 10.1007/s10508-005-7909-6.

Brundu, B., Detaddei, S., Ferdeghini, F., Nappi, R., Polatti, F., & Sommacal, A. (2003). Role of testosterone in feminine sexuality. *Journal of Endocrinological Investigation, 26*(3), 97–101.

Clayton, A. (2010).The pathophysiology of hypoactive sexual desire disorder in women. *International Journal of Gynecology & Obstetrics, 110*(1), 7-11.

Davis, S., & Tran, J. (2001). Testosterone influences libido and well-being in women. *Trends in Endocrinology and Metabolism, 12*(1), 33–37.

Gingell, C., Glasser, D., Laumann, E., Moreira, E., Nicolosi, A., & Wang, T. (2005). Sexual problems among women and men aged 40–80y: Prevalence and correlates identified in the global study of sexual attitudes and behaviors. *International Journal of Impotence Research, 17*(1), 39–57.

Hayes, R., Dennerstein, L., Bennett, C., Koochaki, P., Leiblum, S., & Graziottin, A. (2007). Relationship between hypoactive sexual desire disorder and aging. *Fertil Steril., 87*(1), 107-112.

Hayes, R., Dennerstein, L., Bennett, C., Sidat, M., Gurrin, L., & Fairley, C. K. (2008). Risk factors for female sexual dysfunction in the general population: exploring factors associated with low sexual function and sexual distress. *J Sex Med., 5*(7), 1681-1693.

Hylton, V. J., Chang, C., Sewell, O., Easley, C., Nguyen, C., Dunn, S.,…Beitz, J. (2016). FDA approval of flibanserin — treating hypoactive sexual desire disorder. *N Engl J Med., 374*,101-104. DOI: 10.1056/NEJMp1513686

Irvine, J. (2005). *Disorders of desire*. Philadelphia, PA: Temple University Press.

IsHak, W. W., & Tobia, G. (2013). DSM-5 Changes in Diagnostic Criteria of Sexual Dysfunctions. *Reprod Sys Sexual Disorders, 2*,122. DOI:10.4172/2161-038X.1000122

Kingsberg, S. A. (2011). Hypoactive sexual desire disorder: understanding the impact on midlife women. *The Female Patient, 36*, 1-4.

Lindau, S., Schumm, L. P., Laumann, E. O., Levinson, W., O'Muircheartaigh, C., & Waite, L. (2007). A study of sexuality among older adults in the United States. *N Engl J Med.*, *357*(8), 762–774.

Montgomery, K. A. (2008). Sexual desire disorders. *Psychiatry (Edgmont)*, *5*(6), 50–55.

Nappi, R., Martini, E., Terreno, E., Albani, F., Santamaria, V., Tonani, S.,...Polatti, F. (2010). Management of hypoactive sexual desire disorder in women: current and emerging therapies. *Int J Womens Health*, *2*, 167–175.

Rice, S. C., & Kim, S. K. (2015). *Inhibited sexual desire*. Retrieved from http://www.healthline.com/health/inhibited-sexual-desire#Overview1

Sadock, B. J., & Sadock, V. A. (2003). *Kaplan and Sadock's synopsis of psychiatry: behavioral sciences and clinical psychiatry* (9th ed). Philadelphia, PA: Lippincott Williams & Wilkins.

Shifren, J. L., Monz, B. U., Russo, P., Segreti, A., & Johannes, C. (2008). Sexual problems and distress in United States women: prevalence and correlates. *Obstet Gynecol.*, *112*(5), 970-978.

Stahl, S. (2000). *Essential psychopharmacology: Neuroscientific basis and practical applications*, (2nd ed). New York, NY: Cambridge University Press.

Trudel, G., Marchand, A., Ravart, M., Aubin, S., Turgeon, L., & Fortier, P. (2001). The effect of a cognitive-behavioral group treatment program on hypoactive sexual desire in women. *Sex Relat Ther.*, *16*, 145–164.

Warnock, J. J. (2002). Female hypoactive sexual desire disorder: epidemiology, diagnosis and treatment. *CNS Drugs*, *16*(11), 745-53.

YOUR KNOWLEDGE HAS VALUE

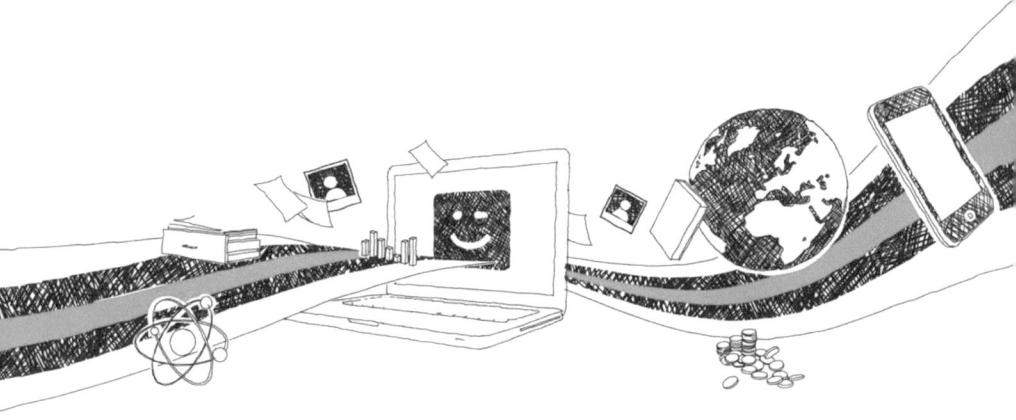

- We will publish your bachelor's and master's thesis, essays and papers

- Your own eBook and book - sold worldwide in all relevant shops

- Earn money with each sale

Upload your text at www.GRIN.com
and publish for free

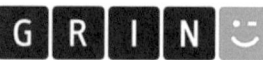